THE ULTIMATE LOW FODMAP DIET COOKBOOK FOR 30-DAYS

"Savoring Wellness One Low FODMAP Recipe at a Time, Discover Delicious Dishes for a Happier Gut and Healthier You"

VICTOR WREN

Copyright © 2023 by Victor Wren

TABLE OF CONTENTS

INTRODUCTION

A. COMPREHENSIVE OVERVIEW OF THE LOW FODMAP DIET

Welcome to "The Definitive Guide to the 30-Day Low FODMAP Diet Cookbook." WIn the forthcoming sections, we will delve into the captivating domain of the Low FODMAP Diet, initially unraveling the essence of FODMAPs. FODMAPs, a shorthand for Fermentable Oligosaccharides, Disaccharides, Monosaccharides, and Polyols, epitomize a category of carbohydrates capable of provoking digestive unease in a multitude of people. This dietary protocol, substantiated by scientific research and warmly adopted by individuals seeking digestive solace, endeavors to lay the foundation for improved health and overall well-being.

B. OBJECTIVES AND AIMS OF THE COOKBOOK

The principal objective of this culinary compendium is to present you with a pragmatic and delectable remedy for the challenges inherent in the Low FODMAP Diet. We understand that embarking on this dietary journey can be daunting, which is why our aim is to provide you with a comprehensive collection of recipes and resources that empower you to effectively follow the diet for a period of 30 days and beyond. By initiating this endeavor, you will be taking a substantial step towards a more joyful and healthier self.

C. EFFECTIVE UTILIZATION OF THIS VOLUME

To maximize the benefits of "The 30-Day Low FODMAP Diet Cookbook: Your Ultimate Guide," it is imperative to understand how to employ this book optimally. Each section has been meticulously crafted to shepherd you through the intricacies of the Low FODMAP Diet, from grasping its fundamental tenets to implementing them in your daily life. With every chapter, you will acquire knowledge, proficiency, and motivation to transform the diet into a pleasurable facet of your existence. Whether you are a neophyte or an individual in search of innovative concepts, there is something here to captivate your interest. The 30-day meal plan serves as your navigational chart to success, teeming with a plethora of delightful recipes to relish during your journey.

Now, let's immerse ourselves in the sections of this cookbook and commence your voyage toward improved digestion and overall well-being.

CHAPTER 1

GRASPING THE ESSENTIALS OF THE LOW FODMAP DIET

A. UNVEILING THE NATURE OF FODMAPs

To embark on a successful journey with the Low FODMAP Diet, it's vital to fathom the essence of this dietary approach. FODMAPs constitute a category of fermentable carbohydrates that are present in a diverse array of foods. The acronym "FODMAP" stands for Fermentable Oligosaccharides, Disaccharides, Monosaccharides, and Polyols. These carbohydrates can be inadequately absorbed in the small intestine, leading to their fermentation in the colon.

This fermentative process can result in the generation of gas, which, in some individuals, may give rise to digestive discomfort, encompassing symptoms such as bloating, flatulence, abdominal pain, and alterations in bowel habits. To mitigate these effects, the Low FODMAP Diet aims to curtail the consumption of high-FODMAP foods and opt for alternatives that are gentler on the digestive system. Understanding which foods are rich or poor in FODMAPs serves as the cornerstone of this diet and underpins our culinary voyage through the ensuing sections.

B. IDENTIFYING BENEFICIARIES OF THE LOW FODMAP DIET

The Low FODMAP Diet has garnered acclaim and recognition for its effectiveness in managing an assortment of gastrointestinal ailments, rendering it a valuable dietary strategy for various demographic groups.

Individuals who can derive advantages from this diet encompass those who:

1. **Encounter irritable bowel syndrome (IBS):** Many individuals grappling with IBS find relief from their symptoms, such as abdominal discomfort, bloating, and erratic bowel movements, by embracing a low FODMAP diet.

2. **Wrestle with inflammatory bowel diseases (IBD):** Individuals afflicted by conditions like Crohn's disease and ulcerative colitis may experience symptom amelioration through the adoption of a low FODMAP approach during periods of exacerbation or unease.

3. **Confront functional gastrointestinal disorders:** Other functional gastrointestinal disorders, like functional dyspepsia, can also derive benefits from this dietary tactic.

It's imperative to recognize that the applicability of a low FODMAP diet is not universal, and its implementation should be overseen by a healthcare professional, dietitian, or medical authority.

C. POTENTIAL HEALTH BENEFITS

Embracing the Low FODMAP Diet unfolds a spectrum of potential health merits transcending the relief of digestive symptoms. These encompass:

1. **Augmented quality of life:** For numerous individuals, the mitigation of digestive discomfort can profoundly enhance their overall well-being and daily existence.

2. **Enhanced dietary consciousness:** The diet fosters a keener understanding of the intricate interplay between nourishment and digestion, leading to more wholesome dietary practices.

3. **Tailored nutrition:** By identifying specific triggers and customizing their diet, individuals can optimize their nutritional intake for enhanced health.

4. **Weight management:** Some individuals find that adhering to a low FODMAP diet can be conducive to achieving their weight management goals.

D. DISPELLING COMMON MISUNDERSTANDINGS

Pervading misconceptions regarding the Low FODMAP Diet are not unusual. Let's address a few of these:

1. **It's a lifelong commitment:** Although the diet may be observed rigorously for a finite period, it is not intended to be a perpetual regimen. The objective is to pinpoint particular triggers and subsequently reintroduce some high-FODMAP foods into your diet.

2. **It's a weight loss diet:** This diet predominantly addresses digestive symptoms, not weight reduction. Weight loss might occur as a consequence of symptom alleviation, but it is not the primary focus.

3. **All high-FODMAP foods are unhealthy:** This is an erroneous assumption. Numerous nutritious foods are abundant in FODMAPs, but they can be constituents of a balanced diet for those not grappling with FODMAP-related issues.

4. **It's excessively restrictive:** While there are some constraints, a well-planned low FODMAP diet can be varied and delectable. This cookbook will facilitate your exploration of an assortment of savory alternatives.

As we delve further into the forthcoming sections, we will debunk additional fallacies and furnish you with the expertise and tools to harness the full potential of the Low FODMAP Diet. Whether you are contemplating this diet for the alleviation of digestive distress or merely seeking a more wholesome rapport with nourishment, comprehending its fundamentals serves as your inaugural stride toward success.

CHAPTER 2

GETTING STARTED

A. PREPARING YOUR KITCHEN

Your kitchen is the heart of your culinary journey on the Low FODMAP Diet. It's where you'll create delicious, digestive-friendly meals. Here's how to prepare your kitchen:

1. **Clear the clutter:** Start by decluttering your pantry, refrigerator, and cabinets. Remove expired or high-FODMAP items that might tempt you.

2. **Stock up on essentials:** Ensure you have essential low FODMAP ingredients like garlic-infused oils, gluten-free flours, and lactose-free dairy alternatives.

3. **Organize your tools:** Make sure your kitchen utensils, measuring cups, and cookware are readily accessible. A few specialty tools like a garlic-infused oil dispenser may also come in handy.

4. **Create a designated FODMAP-friendly zone:** Designate a section of your kitchen for your low FODMAP ingredients. This will help you quickly identify and access suitable foods.

B. GROCERY SHOPPING FOR FODMAP-FRIENDLY INGREDIENTS

A successful Low FODMAP journey starts at the grocery store. Here's how to navigate the aisles:

1. **Expand your knowledge:** Take the time to acquaint yourself with high and low FODMAP foods. Utilize various mobile applications and web-based references to empower yourself with the information needed to make well-informed selections.

2. **Read labels:** Become a label detective. Check ingredient lists for high FODMAP components and opt for suitable alternatives.

3. **Prepare your shopping list:** Prior to your trip to the store, craft a comprehensive list of items aligned with your weekly meal plan. This meticulous planning will assist you in adhering to your dietary objectives.

4. **Select fresh and minimally processed foods:** Opt for fresh produce, lean sources of protein, whole grains, and unprocessed foods. These options are typically naturally low in FODMAPs and serve as healthier choices in comparison to heavily processed alternatives.

C. MEAL PLANNING AND PREPARATION TIPS

Effective meal planning is a cornerstone of the Low FODMAP Diet. Here's how to do it successfully:

1. **Plan ahead:** Set aside time each week to plan your meals. Create a weekly meal schedule, including breakfast, lunch, dinner, and snacks.

2. **Variety is key:** Ensure your meals are diverse and flavorful. Experiment with different low FODMAP ingredients to keep your diet interesting.

3. **Batch cooking:** Save time by preparing large batches of low FODMAP meals and freezing individual portions for later use.

4. **Portion control:** Be mindful of portion sizes. Even low FODMAP foods can become problematic in excessive amounts.

D. DINING OUT AND SOCIAL SITUATIONS

Social situations and dining out can be challenging when following the Low FODMAP Diet. Here's how to navigate these scenarios:

1. **Communicate your needs:** When dining out, don't hesitate to inform the restaurant staff about your dietary requirements. Many restaurants are accommodating and willing to modify dishes.

2. **Plan ahead:** Check restaurant menus online in advance. This allows you to identify potential low FODMAP options and make informed choices.

3. **BYO snacks:** For social events or gatherings, bring your low FODMAP snacks or dishes to ensure you have suitable options.

4. **Educate friends and family:** Share your dietary needs with close friends and family. They can support you by choosing restaurants with low FODMAP options when you dine together.

By preparing your kitchen, mastering grocery shopping, meal planning, and navigating social situations, you'll be well-equipped to embark on a successful 30-day journey with the Low FODMAP Diet. This foundation sets the stage for the delicious recipes and insights we'll explore in the following chapters.

CHAPTER 3

30-DAYS MEAL PLAN

A. WEEK 1: BREAKFAST, LUNCH, AND DINNER RECIPES

Week 1 is your first step into the Low FODMAP Diet journey. In the upcoming week, we will present an array of delectable low FODMAP dishes designed to not only relieve digestive unease but also tantalize your palate. Here's a sneak preview of the culinary offerings in store:

★ **Breakfasts:** Start your day with a hearty and satisfying breakfast. Think of creamy oatmeal topped with fresh berries or a classic omelet filled with spinach and tomatoes.

★ **Lunch:** Lunch options might include a colorful and crisp salad with grilled chicken or a nourishing quinoa bowl loaded with roasted vegetables.

★ **Dinner:** For dinner, enjoy a succulent grilled salmon fillet with a side of garlic-infused mashed potatoes or a comforting bowl of low FODMAP spaghetti with a rich tomato sauce.

B. WEEK 2: BREAKFAST, LUNCH, AND DINNER RECIPES

In Week 2, we'll continue to explore a wide array of low FODMAP recipes, offering you even more variety and culinary excitement. Expect:

★ **Breakfast:** Consider starting your day with a tropical-inspired smoothie or a fluffy stack of gluten-free pancakes.

★ **Lunch:** Embrace a light and fresh caprese salad or indulge in a warm, flavorful chicken stir-fry with low FODMAP veggies.

★ **Dinner:** Dive into a mouthwatering seared steak with rosemary potatoes or savor a bowl of fragrant and aromatic Thai green curry.

C. WEEK 3: BREAKFAST, LUNCH, AND DINNER RECIPES

As you advance into the third week, you'll notice an expansion in your familiarity with low FODMAP components and tastes. Here's a glimpse of what awaits:

★ **Breakfast:** Try a savory breakfast bake with eggs and spinach or a hearty and satisfying chia pudding.

★ **Lunch:** For lunch, explore the flavors of a balsamic-glazed chicken and vegetable wrap or enjoy a fragrant and colorful Mediterranean salad.

★ **Dinner:** Delight in a juicy pork tenderloin with a side of roasted carrots and parsnips or savor the comfort of a hearty beef and vegetable stew.

D. WEEK 4: BREAKFAST, LUNCH, AND DINNER RECIPES

In Week 4, we bring your 30-day Low FODMAP journey to a flavorful conclusion. You've learned to navigate this dietary path with confidence, and now it's time to celebrate your progress:

- ★ **Breakfast:** Round off your breakfast options with a zesty and nutrient-packed green smoothie or a warm bowl of creamy polenta.

- ★ **Lunch:** Enjoy a light and refreshing shrimp and avocado salad or a delicious and hearty turkey and vegetable wrap.

- ★ **Dinner:** As you reach the final week, celebrate with a sumptuous grilled swordfish with lemon herb sauce or a comforting bowl of low FODMAP chili.

This comprehensive 30-day meal plan is crafted to not only bolster your digestive well-being but also kindle your culinary ingenuity. As you explore the subsequent sections, you'll encounter in-depth instructions for each of these meal concepts, accompanied by valuable insights and strategies to transform your Low FODMAP expedition into a pleasurable and scrumptious experience.

CHAPTER 4

DELICIOUS LOW FODMAP RECIPES

A. BREAKFAST OPTIONS

Commence your day with a delectable array of low FODMAP breakfast options. Whether you lean towards a speedy and straightforward morning repast or a leisurely brunch, there's a diverse selection for every palate:

1. **Blueberry Banana Smoothie:** Savor the invigorating fusion of blueberries, banana, lactose-free yogurt, and a touch of maple syrup to enhance your morning.

2. **Feta and Spinach Omelet:** Relish a savory omelet brimming with spinach and lactose-free feta cheese, expertly seasoned for ultimate flavor.

3. **Pancake Stacks:** Fluffy and golden gluten-free pancakes served with a drizzle of maple syrup and fresh strawberries.

B. APPETIZERS AND SNACKS

When you need a quick bite or want to impress guests, these low FODMAP appetizers and snacks have you covered:

1. **Caprese Skewers:** Cherry tomatoes, fresh basil, and mozzarella skewers drizzled with a balsamic glaze.

2. **Quinoa Salad Cups:** Mini quinoa salad cups with diced cucumbers, red bell peppers, and a zesty lemon dressing.

3. **Parmesan Crisps:** Crispy parmesan cheese crisps, perfect for snacking or dipping.

C. MAIN COURSE MEALS

Discover a variety of main course meals that showcase the delicious possibilities of low FODMAP cooking:

1. **Grilled Lemon Herb Chicken:** Succulent chicken breasts marinated in a zesty lemon and herb sauce, served with roasted potatoes.

2. **Salmon with Dill Sauce:** Pan-seared salmon fillets accompanied by a creamy and dairy-free dill sauce.

3. **Asian-Inspired Beef Stir-Fry:** A tantalizing stir-fry featuring thinly sliced beef, colorful bell peppers, and a flavorful low FODMAP sauce.

D. SIDE DISHES

Complement your main courses with delectable low FODMAP side dishes that add depth and variety to your meals:

1. **Roasted Maple Carrots:** Carrot sticks roasted to perfection with a drizzle of maple syrup and a sprinkle of fresh thyme.

2. **Quinoa Pilaf:** Fluffy quinoa mixed with diced zucchini, scallion greens, and a touch of lemon.

3. **Garlic-Infused Mashed Potatoes:** Creamy mashed potatoes made with garlic-infused oil for flavor without the FODMAPs.

E. DESSERTS AND SWEET TREATS

Satisfy your sweet tooth without compromising your low FODMAP journey with these delightful dessert options:

1. **Chocolate-Dipped Strawberries:** Juicy strawberries dipped in dark chocolate for a luscious treat.

2. **Lemon Sorbet:** A refreshing and tangy sorbet made with fresh lemon juice and a touch of sugar.

3. **Almond and Coconut Macaroons:** Chewy and indulgent macaroons made with almond meal and coconut.

These recipes provide a glimpse into the delicious world of low FODMAP cooking. Each dish is thoughtfully crafted to offer not only digestive relief but also an enjoyable culinary experience. In the chapters that follow, you'll find detailed instructions, tips, and variations for these and many more mouthwatering recipes.

CHAPTER 5

MANAGING NUTRITIONAL NEEDS

A. BALANCING YOUR DIET

Sustaining a well-rounded diet is crucial for your holistic well-being, even as you adhere to the Low FODMAP Diet. Here's how to guarantee that your nutritional requisites are fulfilled:

1. **Diversity:** Integrate an extensive spectrum of low FODMAP foods to secure a rich assortment of nutrients. Rotate your ingredients to evade repetitiveness and capitalize on an array of vitamins and minerals.

2. **Food Groups:** Aim to include foods from various food groups, such as fruits, vegetables, proteins, and grains. This ensures a well-rounded diet.

3. **Micronutrients:** Give due consideration to vital micronutrients, including vitamins and minerals. It's advisable to seek guidance from a registered dietitian to confirm that you are fulfilling your distinct nutritional needs.

B. NUTRIENT-RICH FODMAP-FRIENDLY FOODS

While adhering to a low FODMAP dietary regimen, you have the opportunity to relish an extensive array of nutrient-dense foods:

1. **Low FODMAP Fruits:** Embrace fruits such as strawberries, kiwi, and oranges that not only boast low FODMAP content but also offer a wealth of vitamin C and antioxidants to fortify your health.

2. **Low FODMAP Vegetables:** Include vegetables like spinach, carrots, and bell peppers in your meals, as they deliver vital vitamins and fiber to enhance your overall nutrition.

3. **Protein Sources:** Opt for lean protein sources such as chicken, turkey, fish, and tofu. Not only are these selections low in FODMAPs, but they also provide high-quality protein for sustained energy and muscular well-being.

4. **Grains:** Relish gluten-free grains like rice, quinoa, and oats, infusing your dishes with dietary fiber and a diverse array of essential nutrients.

5. **Lactose-Free Dairy:** Elect lactose-free dairy products or dairy alternatives enriched with calcium and vitamin D to bolster your bone health.

6. **Nuts and Seeds:** Snack on low FODMAP nuts like almonds and macadamia nuts, which offer healthy fats and protein.

It's important to note that despite the restrictions of the Low FODMAP Diet, you can still consume a nutritionally rich diet by selecting suitable alternatives within each food group.

C. PORTION CONTROL

Portion control plays a crucial role in managing the Low FODMAP Diet:

1. **Serving Sizes:** Be mindful of recommended serving sizes for low FODMAP foods. Consuming large quantities of certain ingredients may lead to higher FODMAP intake.

2. **Balanced Plates:** Aim for balanced meals with appropriate portions of protein, carbohydrates, and vegetables. This helps prevent overconsumption of high FODMAP ingredients.

3. **Snacking:** If you find yourself snacking frequently, choose low FODMAP options and control portion sizes. Pre-portioning snacks can be a helpful strategy.

4. **Hydration:** Remember the importance of staying well-hydrated. Water is essential for digestion and overall health. Sip water throughout the day to maintain proper hydration.

Throughout your 30-day Low FODMAP expedition, ensuring equilibrium in your dietary choices, selecting foods abundant in essential nutrients, and mastering portion management will be instrumental in sustaining a nutritionally robust meal strategy that bolsters your overall health. Striking a harmonious equilibrium in your nutritional requirements is pivotal in attaining both digestive solace and peak well-being.

CHAPTER 6

DEALING WITH CHALLENGES

A. COPING WITH FOOD CRAVINGS

One of the prevalent hurdles encountered while following the Low FODMAP Diet is handling food desires, particularly when you experience an intense yearning for high FODMAP fare. Here's how to effectively deal with these situations:

1. **Substitute Smartly:** Identify suitable low FODMAP alternatives for your favorite high FODMAP foods. For example, if you crave garlic, use garlic-infused oil for a similar flavor.

2. **Practice Mindfulness:** When cravings strike, pause and ask yourself if you're genuinely hungry or just experiencing a craving. Mindful eating can help you make better choices.

3. **Stay Prepared:** Keep low FODMAP snacks on hand to curb cravings. Snack options like mixed nuts, hard cheeses, and rice cakes can satisfy your taste buds.

B. OVERCOMING DINING-OUT DILEMMAS

Dining out while following a low FODMAP diet can be challenging, but it's not impossible. Here's how to navigate restaurant meals:

1. **Plan Ahead:** Research the restaurant's menu online before going out. Look for dishes that are likely to be low FODMAP or can be modified.

2. **Communicate Clearly:** Don't hesitate to inform the waiter about your dietary requirements. Request modifications or substitutions to make dishes suitable for you.

3. **BYO Sauce:** Carry small bottles of condiments like garlic-infused oil or your preferred low FODMAP sauce. This way, you can add flavor to your meal while dining out.

C. NAVIGATING SOCIAL EVENTS

Social events and gatherings can be tricky when following a low FODMAP diet. Here's how to handle these situations:

1. **Inform Your Host:** If you're attending an event at someone's home, politely inform your host about your dietary needs. They may be willing to accommodate you.

2. **BYO Dish:** When appropriate, bring a low FODMAP dish to share with others. This ensures you have something safe to eat and introduces others to delicious low FODMAP options.

3. **Eat Beforehand:** If you're uncertain about the food options at an event, eat a small meal or snack before attending, so you're not overly hungry and less likely to be tempted by high FODMAP offerings.

4. **Focus on Socializing**: At social events, shift the focus from food to socializing. Engage in conversations, games, or activities to minimize the emphasis on eating.

Dealing with challenges, cravings, dining-out dilemmas, and social events requires a combination of planning, communication, and a positive mindset. By employing these strategies, you can successfully navigate various scenarios while maintaining your commitment to the Low FODMAP Diet.

CHAPTER 7

SUCCESS STORIES AND TESTIMONIALS

A. Real-Life Experiences of Individuals on the Low FODMAP Diet

Within this section, we will immerse ourselves in the genuine life encounters of individuals who have initiated their journey on the Low FODMAP Diet. These personal accounts encapsulate the trials, victories, and conversions that transpire during the course of this dietary expedition. By revealing their narratives, our intention is to ignite inspiration and extend a sense of fellowship to those who might be treading a parallel route.

★ **Case Study: Sarah's Digestive Relief:** Meet Sarah, a young professional who had struggled with IBS for years. Through her commitment to the Low FODMAP Diet, she experienced a dramatic reduction in her symptoms, allowing her to enjoy life without the constant discomfort.

★ **Interview with Mark:** Mark, an athlete and fitness enthusiast, shares how he optimized his diet on the Low FODMAP plan. His story demonstrates how this diet can be tailored to support various lifestyles, including those with active fitness routines.

★ **Family Success**: The Smith family's journey showcases the adaptability of the Low FODMAP Diet. Their collective effort to support a family member with IBS led to healthier eating habits for the entire family, strengthening their bonds and overall well-being.

B. INSPIRATIONAL STORIES

Beyond the trials and triumphs, inspirational stories demonstrate the incredible impact of the Low FODMAP Diet on individuals' lives. These stories highlight the resilience, optimism, and transformation that can result from embracing this dietary approach.

★ **Mary's Journey to Wellness:** Mary, a teacher and mother of two, shares her story of resilience and determination. Her journey from frequent discomfort to improved health through the Low FODMAP Diet is a testament to the power of positive change.

★ **Finding Freedom Through Food:** James, a musician who often travels for work, narrates his inspiring story of discovering dietary freedom and control. He found that by mastering the Low FODMAP Diet, he could pursue his passion for music without digestive disruptions.

★ **Liz's Remarkable Journey:** Liz's evolution from the constraints imposed by her digestive complications to a life filled with vitality and activity serves as an inspiring illustration of how the Low FODMAP Diet can embolden individuals to seize control of their well-being and chase after their aspirations.

These accounts of triumph and motivating narratives serve as poignant reminders that the Low FODMAP Diet represents more than a mere nutritional plan; it is a gateway to a life marked by enhanced health, contentment, and fulfillment. They stand as shining lights of optimism and incentive for anyone endeavoring to enhance their digestive health and overall quality of life.

CHAPTER 8

FAQ AND TROUBLESHOOTING

A. COMMON QUESTIONS AND CONCERNS

This chapter addresses some of the most common questions and concerns that individuals following the Low FODMAP Diet often encounter. By providing clear and informative answers, we aim to offer guidance and alleviate uncertainties:

1. **"Is the Low FODMAP Diet suitable for everyone?":** Explore the criteria for determining if this diet is appropriate for various individuals.

2. **"Can I ever reintroduce high FODMAP foods?":** Understand the process of food reintroduction and how it can expand your dietary choices.

3. **"How long should I follow the Low FODMAP Diet?":** Learn about the recommended duration and potential long-term modifications.

4. **"Will I miss out on important nutrients?":** Address concerns about nutrient deficiencies and strategies for maintaining a balanced diet.

5. **"What if I have dietary restrictions or preferences?":** Discover how to adapt the Low FODMAP Diet to accommodate vegetarian, vegan, or gluten-free preferences.

B. PRACTICAL SOLUTIONS TO COMMON ISSUES

When following a specialized diet like the Low FODMAP Diet, challenges are bound to arise. This section provides practical solutions to help readers overcome these issues:

1. **Managing Travel:** Tips for maintaining your diet while traveling, including packing snacks, researching restaurant options, and being prepared for different culinary experiences.

2. **Dealing with Stress:** Strategies for minimizing the impact of stress on your digestive health, such as mindfulness practices, exercise, and relaxation techniques.

3. **Balancing Fiber Intake:** Recommendations for maintaining adequate fiber while on a low FODMAP diet, including suitable sources and portion control.

4. **Budget-Friendly Options:** Ideas for keeping your Low FODMAP journey cost-effective, such as buying in bulk, meal planning, and making use of budget-friendly ingredients.

5. **Coping with Setbacks:** Guidance for handling setbacks, including understanding triggers, reevaluating your diet, and regaining control.

By addressing common questions and concerns while providing practical solutions to everyday challenges, this chapter equips readers with the knowledge and tools they need to successfully navigate the Low FODMAP Diet, maintaining their health and well-being.

CONCLUSION

A. RECAP OF THE 30-DAYS JOURNEY

Congratulations on completing **"The Ultimate Low FODMAP Diet Cookbook for 30 Days"**! Over the past month, you've embarked on a transformative journey to better digestive health and culinary exploration. Let's take a moment to reflect on your achievements:

You started by understanding what FODMAPs are and who can benefit from this diet. You delved into the essentials of low FODMAP living, from preparing your kitchen to dining out with confidence. You experienced the diverse flavors of a 30-day meal plan and discovered how nutrient-rich foods can support your well-being. You learned how to overcome challenges, deal with cravings, and navigate social situations.

B. THE ROAD AHEAD: Maintaining a Low FODMAP Lifestyle

As you wrap up this month-long odyssey, it's pivotal to contemplate the path that lies ahead. Sustaining a low FODMAP way of life entails not only the knowledge you've acquired but also the manner in which you consistently integrate it into your everyday existence:

1. **Reintroduction:** Consider the next phase of your journey – reintroducing high FODMAP foods. This can help you identify your personal triggers and expand your dietary choices.

2. **Sustainability:** Embrace the Low FODMAP Diet as a long-term lifestyle rather than a short-term solution. Continue to prioritize low FODMAP foods, adapt recipes, and enjoy the benefits of a happier digestive system.

3. **Personalization:** Customize your low FODMAP lifestyle to fit your individual needs. Experiment with different ingredients, explore international cuisines, and create a diet that works best for you.

C. ADDITIONAL RESOURCES AND REFERENCES

To further support your low FODMAP journey, here are some additional resources and references to explore:

1. **Consult a Dietitian:** A registered dietitian with expertise in the Low FODMAP Diet can provide personalized guidance and recommendations.

2. **Online Communities:** Connect with others on a similar path by joining online communities and forums where you can share experiences, recipes, and tips.

3. **Cookbooks:** Explore more cookbooks and resources dedicated to low FODMAP cooking to keep your culinary creativity thriving.

4. **Healthcare Experts:** Uphold transparent and ongoing communication with your medical practitioner to oversee your digestive health and seek counsel when necessary.

Recall, this voyage extends beyond the contents of your plate; it encompasses your comprehensive well-being. The wisdom and competencies you've amassed during this 30-day encounter will remain your steadfast companions as you proceed. Incorporate the delectable low FODMAP recipes from this cookbook into your culinary repertoire, and savor a life characterized by reduced digestive inconveniences and augmented joy with every meal. Your route to well-being and felicity genuinely rests within your control, and you've embarked on the inaugural stages toward a more radiant and agreeable future.

APPENDICES

A. LOW FODMAP FOOD LISTS

Within this division, you will encounter exhaustive inventories of low FODMAP comestibles, which will aid you in making well-considered selections for your repasts. These enumerations are categorized by food type, streamlining the process of pinpointing fitting components for your culinary creations and dietary inclinations.

- ➤ **Fruits:** Discover low FODMAP fruit options, from berries to citrus fruits, that can add natural sweetness to your diet.

- ➤ **Vegetables:** Explore a wide array of low FODMAP vegetables to create colorful and nutritious dishes.

- ➤ **Proteins:** Find sources of lean proteins that align with your low FODMAP lifestyle, from poultry to tofu.

➢ **Grains:** Identify gluten-free grains that can serve as the foundation for satisfying meals.

➢ **Dairy and Alternatives:** Learn about lactose-free dairy products and dairy alternatives suitable for your dietary needs.

➢ **Nuts and Seeds:** Discover low FODMAP options for snacking and incorporating into your recipes.

B. PRINTABLE MEAL PLANNING WORKSHEETS

For enhanced convenience and increased efficiency in meal preparation, we've furnished printable meal planning templates that are at your disposal for structuring your daily and weekly meals. These templates encompass sections designated for breakfast, lunch, dinner, and snacks, affording you the means to chart your 30-day expedition.

➢ **Daily Meal Planner:** Plan your meals for the day, noting specific recipes and portion sizes.

> **Weekly Meal Planner:** Organize your week's meals in advance, ensuring variety and balance.

> **Shopping List:** Create a shopping list based on your meal plans, making grocery shopping a breeze.

> **Progress Tracker:** Keep track of your dietary journey, noting any observations, symptoms, or reactions.

C. RECIPE INDEX

The recipe index is a handy reference to quickly locate specific recipes within this cookbook. It lists recipes by category, making it simple to find your favorite low FODMAP dishes or explore new ones:

> **Breakfast Options:** Find your preferred morning meal, from smoothies to omelets.

> **Appetizers and Snacks:** Discover quick and delicious starters and snacks for any occasion.

> **Main Course Meals:** Browse through a wide selection of satisfying main courses, from poultry to seafood.

> **Side Dishes:** Complement your meals with flavorful and nutritious side dishes.

> **Desserts and Sweet Treats:** Satisfy your sweet tooth with mouthwatering dessert options.

The appendices in this book serve as valuable resources for your continued low FODMAP journey. You'll find the information and tools you need to maintain your dietary success, stay organized, and explore a world of delicious recipes while keeping digestive discomfort at bay.

ACKNOWLEDGMENTS

I extend my heartfelt gratitude to the many individuals who made "The Ultimate Low FODMAP Diet Cookbook for 30 Days" possible. Your contributions, testing, and unwavering support have been instrumental in bringing this cookbook to life.

THANKING CONTRIBUTORS, TESTERS, AND SUPPORTERS

★ **Contributors:** To those who generously shared their expertise, recipes, and insights, your valuable input has enriched this cookbook and provided readers with a diverse range of culinary delights.

★ **Testers:** A heartfelt thank you to all the dedicated recipe testers who meticulously tried and reviewed each dish. Your feedback ensured that the recipes were not only delicious but also reliable for our readers.

★ **Champions:** To each of the friends, family members, and advocates who provided unwavering encouragement and kindled motivation during this creative odyssey, your faith in this undertaking was the propelling energy that brought it to fruition.

This cookbook stands as a tribute to the potential of cooperation, unwavering commitment, and a mutual ardor for delectable cuisine.

I extend my heartfelt gratitude for your priceless input, and my wish is that this book functions as a wellspring of motivation and gastronomic delight for all those embarking on the Low FODMAP Diet.

THE END